もう焦らない!!

英語で伝える検査手順

Jeremy Williams 著
小島 多香子

胸部X線写真撮影編

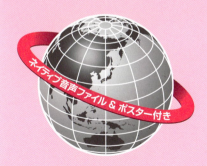

ネイティブ音声ファイル & ポスター付き

医歯薬出版株式会社

This book was originally published in Japanese
under the title of :

EIGO DE TSUTAERU KENSATEJUN — KYOUBU X-SEN SHASHIN SATSUEI HEN
(Taking a chest X-ray)

Authors ;
WILLIAMS, Jeremy
Professor and Chairman, Department of International Medical Communications,
Tokyo Medical University

KOJIMA, Takako
Assistant Professor, Department of International Medical Communications,
Tokyo Medical University

© 2018   1st ed.

ISHIYAKU PUBLISHERS, INC.
  7-10, Honkomagome 1 chome, Bunkyo-ku,
  Tokyo 113-8612, Japan

はじめに

　みなさんは，外国で病院にかかったことはありますか？

　病気やけがをしたときに，言葉の通じない病院でのやりとりは不安がつのるばかりです．またその状況は患者さんだけではなく，迅速かつ適切な対応を求められる医療スタッフにとっても心もとないものです．

　昨年出版しました「もう焦らない！！　英語で伝える検査手順―採血編」と「採尿編」は，必要最低限の英語表現で対応できるようになりたい皆さんのためにまとめたものです．

　本書では，引き続き第3弾として「胸部X線写真撮影」を取り上げてみました．

　検査手順の流れに沿って，より専門的な英語表現を収録しましたので，学習ツールとしてだけではなく，実用書として職場でも活用いただければと思います．

　ぜひ本書で身につけた英語表現で，外国人の患者さんと気軽にコミュニケーションをとり，今後ますますのご活躍ができますことをお祈り申し上げます．

2018年1月

ジェレミー・ウィリアムス
小島多香子

CONTENTS

はじめに ……………………………………………………… iii

音声データのダウンロード ……………………………………… vi

レッスン編

リスニング ……………………………………………………… 2

会　話 …………………………………………………………… 6

練　習 …………………………………………………………… 14

撮影手順の応用場面編

● カルテ受付 ……………………………………………… 16

　患者さんの確認 ………………………………………… 17

　【患者さんが女性の場合】……………………………… 18

　撮影前……………………………………………………… 19

● 撮　　影

撮影（1） ……………………………………… **22**

撮影（2） ……………………………………… **23**

他の一般的な撮影：腕 ………………………… **24**

他の一般的な撮影：足 ………………………… **25**

● 撮影終了 ……………………………………… **32**

診療科の英語表記 ………………………… **36**

解　答 ……………………………………… **38**

執筆者・執筆協力者 ……………………… **41**

音声データのダウンロード

https://www.ishiyaku.co.jp/ebooks/731810/

本書の音声データ（音声マークが付いている部分）を，上記アドレスから無料でダウンロードすることができます．

※再生にはMP3形式の音声データを
再生できるプレイヤーが必要です．

お問い合わせは以下のフォームよりお願いいたします．
https://www.ishiyaku.co.jp/ebooks/inquiry/

レッスン編

＊解答は38頁

リスニング
Listening Practice

Step 1 (Track 1)

これから聞こえる言葉やフレーズを，声を出して繰り返して言ってみましょう．
意味がわからなくても，発音に注意して聞いてみましょう．

Step 2 (Track 2)

次の言葉を聞こえてくる順番に番号をつけましょう．

- robe (　　　)
- shoulders (　　　)
- anti-clockwise (　　　)
- rest (　　　)
- hold (　　　)
- palm (　　　)
- hips (　　　)
- chin (　　　)
- clockwise (　　　)
- roll forward (　　　)
- changing room (　　　)
- hold your breath (　　　)
- metal objects (　　　)

Step 3

ここで単語リスト(Vocabulary List)を覚えましょう.
すべて覚えられなくても心配はいりません.これから行うリスニングの練習で必ず身につきます.

date of birth	生年月日
changing room	更衣室
robe	ガウン(検査着)
shoulders	肩
roll forward	前方に動かす
leave	そのままにする
chin rest	あごを載せる台
hips	腰
hold your breath	息を止める
breathe out	息を吐く
breathe in	息を吸う
palm	手のひら
clockwise	時計回り
anti-clockwise	反時計回り
metal objects	金属類

Step 4

英語の言葉やフレーズと同じ意味の日本語を選び，線で結びましょう．

clockwise	・	・前方に動かす
chin	・	・ガウン（検査着）
changing room	・	・反時計回り
robe	・	・金属性のもの
hold	・	・腰
shoulders	・	・手のひら
metal objects	・	・更衣室
hips	・	・止める
roll forward	・	・時計回り
palm	・	・肩
anti-clockwise	・	・あご

Step 5 (Track 3)

これから聞こえる音声をよく聞いて，その単語や英文を記入しましょう．

1.
2.
3.
4.
5.
6.

7.

8.

9.

10.

Step 6 (Track 4)

これから聞こえる日本語の言葉やフレーズと同じ意味の英語を記入してみましょう．

1.

2.

3.

4.

5.

6.

7.

8.

9.

10.

会 話
Dialog

次の会話を聞きましょう．できれば、繰り返し聞きましょう．しかし，覚える必要はありません．ここで大事なことは，英語に耳を慣らすことです．

診療放射線技師 Medical radiology technician は，
英文表記では "MRT"，日本語表記では「技師」と略しています．

Step 1 (Track 5)
Confirming the patient's identity　患者さんの確認

MRT　　：Please let me confirm your name and date of birth.
Patient：Yes, I'm John Smith, and I was born on June 6, 1972.

【 *For female patients* 】

MRT　　：Are you pregnant, or do you think you might be pregnant?

Step 2 (Track 6)
Getting the patient ready　患者さんの撮影準備

MRT　　：We are going to take a chest X-ray.
　　　　　　We need to take two: one from the front and one from the side, OK?
Patient：OK, no problem.

* 各会話では次のような練習を順番に行います

1）英語の会話を聞きます
2）英語の質問を繰り返し言いましょう
3）「日本語で○○は何と言いますか？」の後に，英語で適切な質問を言いましょう

技　師：確認のためお名前と生年月日を教えてください．
患　者：はい．ジョン・スミスです．1972年6月6日生まれです．

【患者さんが女性の場合】
技　師：妊娠していますか，または妊娠している可能性はありますか？

技　師：これから胸部 X 線写真を撮影します．
　　　　正面と側方の2つの方向から撮影する必要があります．
　　　　よろしいですか？
患　者：はい，わかりました．

MRT : Please step this way. Here is the changing room. Please change into the robe provided. Be careful to remove any metal objects you might be wearing, such as a ring or pendant.

Patient : Can I leave them in the basket?

MRT : Yes, that's fine. Just go through that door when you are ready.

Step 3 (Track 7)
Taking the X-ray 1　X線写真撮影（1）

MRT : First, we are going to take a front X-ray. Please place your chin on the rest, here.

Patient : Here?

MRT : Yes, that's right. Now, place your chest against the plate, here.

Patient : Like this?

MRT : OK, now roll your shoulders forward, （患者さんの姿勢を調整しながら）That's fine.

Step 4 (Track 8)
Depending on physical capability of patient
患者さんの身体的能力によっては

MRT : Rest your hands on your hips like this.

　　　　　　もしくは

Just hold the sides of the plate with your hands, like this.

技　師：こちらへおいでください．更衣室で用意されている検査着に着替えてください．
　　　　また，指輪やペンダントなど身に付けている金属類ははずしてください．
患　者：服はカゴに置いたままでいいですか？
技　師：はい，いいですよ．準備ができたなら，そのドアからお入りください．

技　師：はじめに正面を撮影します．あごを台にのせてください．

患　者：ここですか？
技　師：そうです．そして，胸をこちらのプレートにつけてください．

患　者：こうですか？
技　師：はい．そこで，肩を前方に動かしてください．
　　　　（患者さんの姿勢を調整しながら）そこでいいです．

技　師：このように手を自分のお尻の上に載せてください．
　　　　　　　　　もしくは
　　　　このように，プレートの側面に手を置いてください．

Step 5 (Track 9) Taking the X-ray 2
X線写真撮影（2）

MRT : OK, now take a deep breath and hold. Don't move; it will only take a second.
OK, you can breathe out now.

Patient : Can I get changed now?

MRT : No, not yet. We have to take one more from the side.

Patient : OK.

MRT : Right, now place the right side of your chest against the plate.

   もしくは

now place the left side of your chest against the plate.
Breathe in and hold until I say.
OK, we have finished.

Patient : Can I get changed now?

MRT : Yes, that's fine. Goodbye.

Patient : Thank you.

Step 6 (Track 10) Other common X-rays: the arm
他の一般的な撮影：腕

MRT : OK, now rest your arm here with the palm facing up.

   もしくは

技　師	：では，深く息を吸って，止めて動かないでください．
	すぐ終わります．はい，息を吐いていいですよ．

患　者	：もう着替えてもいいですか？
技　師	：いいえ，もう1枚を側方から撮らなければなりません．

患　者	：わかりました．
技　師	：では，右胸をこちらのプレートに付けてください．

　　　　　　もしくは
　　　　左胸をこちらのプレートに付けてください．

　　　　私がいいと言うまで，息を吸い込んで止めてください．
　　　　はい，終わりました．

患　者	：もう着替えてもいいですか？
技　師	：はい，いいですよ．さようなら．
患　者	：ありがとうございました．

技　師	：では，手のひらを上に向けて，ここに腕を載せてください．

　　　　　　もしくは

OK, now rest your arm here with the palm facing down.

Patient ： Like this?

MRT ： Yes, now just rotate your arm clockwise.

   もしくは

now just rotate your arm anti-clockwise.

OK, stop. Please hold still.

Step 7 (Track 11) Other common X-rays: the leg
他の一般的な撮影：足

MRT ： OK, please lie here, face down.

   もしくは

OK, please lie here, face up.

（姿勢を調整しながら）

OK, now just hold until I say you can move.

Patient ： OK.

MRT ： OK, we are going to take one more.

Please lie down on your left side.

   もしくは

Please lie down on your right side.

では，手のひらを下に向けて，ここに腕を載せてください．

患　者：このように？
技　師：そうです．時計回りに，腕を回してください．
　　　　　　　もしくは
　　　　反時計回りに，腕を回してください．
　　　　そこで止めてください．そのままですよ．

技　師：うつぶせになってください．
　　　　　　　もしくは
　　　　はい，仰向けになってください．

　　　　私が動いていいですよと言うまで，姿勢を保ってください．
患　者：はい．
技　師：それでは，もう1枚を撮りますね．
　　　　あなたの左側を下にしてください．
　　　　　　　もしくは
　　　　あなたの右側を下にしてください．

練 習
Practice

Track 12

次の文章を聞いて，空欄に記入しましょう．

a) Here is the _____.

b) Just _____ forward.

c) Can I _____ in the basket?

d) Let me confirm your _____.

e) Take a _____.

f) _____ your arm here with the _____.

g) _____ your arm _____.

h) Rest your hands _____.

i) Please _____ the robe provided.

j) You can _____ now.

k) Can I _____ now?

撮影手順の
応用場面編

＊レッスン編の会話で示した例文とは異なる場合もあります

胸部Ｘ写真撮影編

● カルテ受付

カルテをお預かりします．

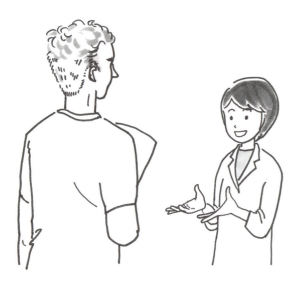

May I have your chart, please?

確認のためお名前と生年月日を教えてください．
お名前はフルネームでお願いします．

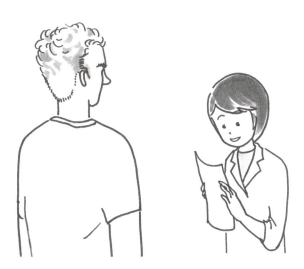

Please let me confirm your name and date of birth. Can you give me your full name?

【患者さんが女性の場合】

妊娠していますか，または妊娠している可能性はありますか？

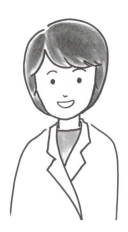

Are you pregnant, or do you think you might be pregnant?

これから胸の写真を
正面と横の2枚，撮影します．

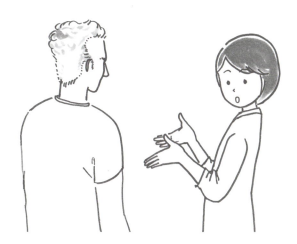

撮影手順の応用場面編

**We are going to take a chest X-ray.
We need to take two: one from
the front and one from the side, OK?**

胸部 X 写真撮影編

こちらの更衣室で，この検査着に着替えてください．
また，指輪やペンダントなどの金属類ははずしてください．

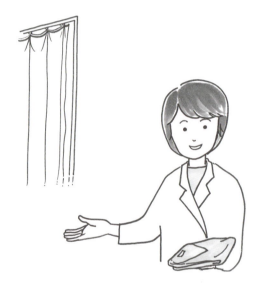

**Please change into the robe provided in the changing room.
Be careful to remove any metal objects you might be wearing, such as a ring or pendant.**

着替えが済みましたら撮影室へ入ってください.

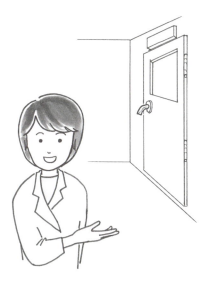

Just go through that door when you are ready.

胸部X写真撮影編

● 撮　影

それではこちらへ．（と撮影装置の方へ誘導する）

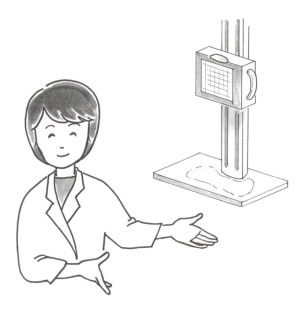

Please step this way.

はじめに正面の撮影をします．

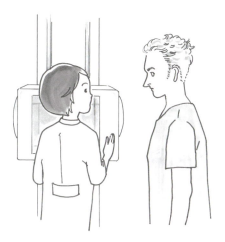

First, we are going to take a front X-ray.

胸部X写真撮影編

あごをこちらにのせ,
胸をこちらのプレートにつけてください.

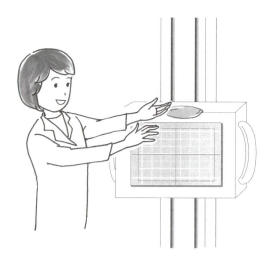

**Please place your chin on the rest here,
and place your chest against the plate.**

両腕はこのようにしてください.

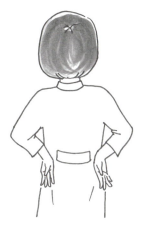

※肩甲骨を開きます

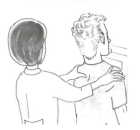

Place your arms here, like this.

深く息を吸って，止めて動かないでください．

→撮　影

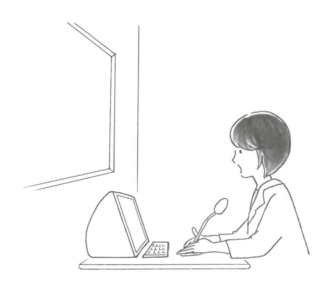

**Now take a deep breath and hold.
Don't move until I say.**

はい，終わりました．

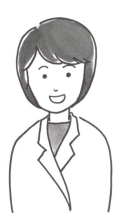

OK, we have finished.

では次に横向きを撮影します.

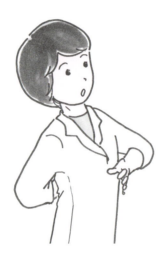

We have to take one more from the side.

左胸を
こちらのプレートにつけてください．

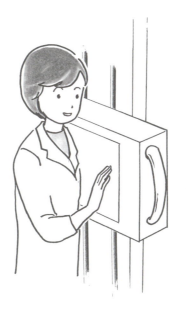

**Now place the left side of
your chest against the plate.**

撮影手順の応用場面編

このバーを持ってください.

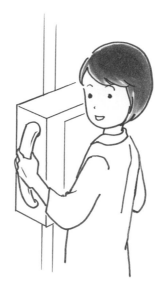

Hold onto this bar.

息を吸って，止めて動かないでください．

→撮　影

撮影手順の応用場面編

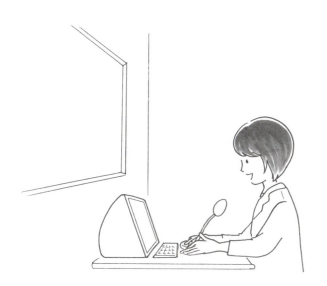

Breathe in and hold until I say.

●撮影終了

これで撮影は終わりです．着替えてください．

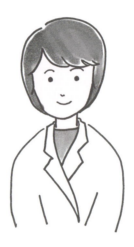

OK, we have finished.
You can change back into your clothes now.

忘れ物のないように荷物を確認ください．

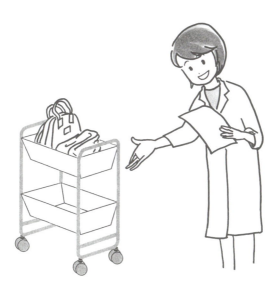

Please make sure you have all your belongings.

撮影手順の応用場面編

カルテをお返しいたします．

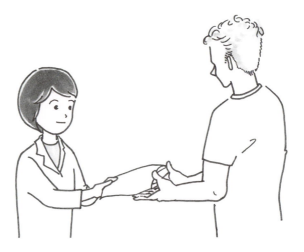

Here is your chart.

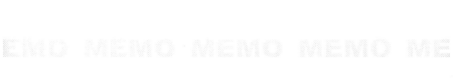

診療科の英語表記

総合診療科　General Medicine and Primary Care
循環器内科　Cardiology
呼吸器内科　Respiratory Medicine
消化器内科　Gastroenterology
腎臓内科　Nephrology
糖尿病・代謝・内分泌内科　Diabetes, Metabolism, Endocrinology
血液内科　Hematology Medicine
感染症科　Infectious Diseases
神経内科　Neurology
高齢診療科　Geriatric Medicine
メンタルヘルス科　Mental Health Medicine
小児科　Pediatrics
リウマチ・膠原病内科　Rheumatology, Collagen Diseases
呼吸器外科・甲状腺外科　Respiratory Tract, Thyroid Surgery
心臓血管外科　Cardiovascular Surgery
消化器外科　Digestive Surgery
小児外科　Pediatric Surgery
脳神経外科　Neurosurgery
整形外科　Orthopedic Surgery
乳腺科　Breast Surgery
麻酔科　Anesthesiology
泌尿器科　Urology
臨床腫瘍科　Medical Oncology
産科・婦人科　Obstetrics and Gynecology
皮膚科　Dermatology

眼科　Ophthalmology
耳鼻咽喉科　Otorhinolaryngology
精神医学　Psychiatry
放射線科　Radiology
形成外科　Plastic and Reconstructive Surgery
歯科口腔外科・矯正歯科　Oral-Maxillofacial Surgery, Dentistry and Orthodontics
病理診断科　Diagnostic Pathology
臨床検査医学科　Laboratory Medicine

レッスン編　解答

【Track 2】解　答

robe (	8	)	shoulders (	7)
anti-clockwise (	6	)	rest (	10)
hold (	2	)	palm (	12)
hips (	3	)	chin (	1)
clockwise (	5	)	roll forward (	4)
changing room (	9	)	hold your breath (	11)
metal objects (	13	)		

【Track 3】解　答

1. Rest your hands on your hips like this.
2. Hold your breath.
3. Please change into the robe provided.
4. Breathe out.
5. Take a deep breath and hold.
6. Place your chest against the plate.
7. Rest your arm here with the palm facing up.
8. Rotate your arm clockwise.
9. Place your chin on the rest.
10. Be careful to remove any metal objects you might be wearing.

【Track 4】解　答

1. Place your chin on the rest.

2. Be careful to remove any metal objects you might be wearing.
3. Please change into the robe provided.
4. Place your chest against the plate.
5. Rest your hands on your hips like this.
6. Hold your breath.
7. Take a deep breath and hold.
8. Rest your arm here with the palm facing up.
9. Rotate your arm clockwise.
10. Breathe out.

> ※ Track 4 の出題音声は「～してください」とありますが，英文表記では，「Please」を付ける必要はかならずしもありません．

【Track 12】解　答

a) Here is the changing room.
b) Just roll your shoulders forward.
c) Can I leave them in the basket?
d) Let me confirm your name.
e) Take a deep breath.
f) Rest your arm here with the palm facing up.
g) Rotate your arm clockwise.
h) Rest your hands on your hips.
i) Please change into the robe provided.
j) You can breathe out now.
k) Can I get changed now?

謝　辞

　本書の執筆において，ご協力およびご助言をいただきました，東京医科大学国際医学情報学分野の高野秀子氏に感謝申し上げます．

執筆者・執筆協力者

【執筆者】

Jeremy Williams（ジェレミー ウイリアムス）　（東京医科大学主任教授　国際医学情報分野）

小島　多香子（こじま　たかこ）（東京医科大学講師　国際医学情報分野）

【執筆協力者】

後藤　多津子（ごとう　たづこ）（東京歯科大学教授　歯科放射線学講座）

井上　孝（いのうえ　たかし）（東京歯科大学教授　同大学千葉病院臨床検査部長）

【イラスト】

Indy yutaka

もう焦らない!! 英語で伝える検査手順
——胸部X線写真撮影編　　ISBN978-4-263-73181-9

2018年1月10日　第1版第1刷発行

著　者　Jeremy Williams
　　　　小　島　多香子
発行者　白　石　泰　夫
発行所　医歯薬出版株式会社

〒113-8612　東京都文京区本駒込1-7-10
TEL. (03)5395-7640(編集)・7616(販売)
FAX. (03)5395-7624(編集)・8563(販売)
https://www.ishiyaku.co.jp/
郵便振替番号　00190-5-13816

乱丁,落丁の際はお取り替えいたします　　印刷・教文堂／製本・愛千製本所
© Ishiyaku Publishers, Inc., 2018. Printed in Japan

本書の複製権・翻訳権・翻案権・上映権・譲渡権・貸与権・公衆送信権（送信可能化権を含む）・口述権は，医歯薬出版㈱が保有します．
本書を無断で複製する行為（コピー，スキャン，デジタルデータ化など）は，「私的使用のための複製」などの著作権法上の限られた例外を除き禁じられています．また私的使用に該当する場合であっても，請負業者等の第三者に依頼し上記の行為を行うことは違法となります．

JCOPY ＜㈳出版者著作権管理機構　委託出版物＞
本書をコピーやスキャン等により複製される場合は，そのつど事前に㈳出版者著作権管理機構(電話 03-3513-6969, FAX 03-3513-6979, e-mail：info@jcopy.or.jp)の許諾を得てください．

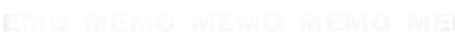

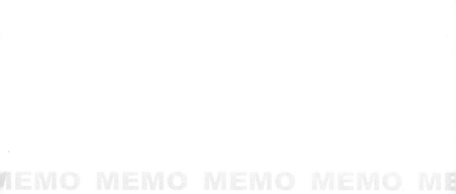

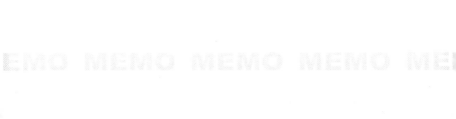

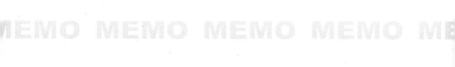